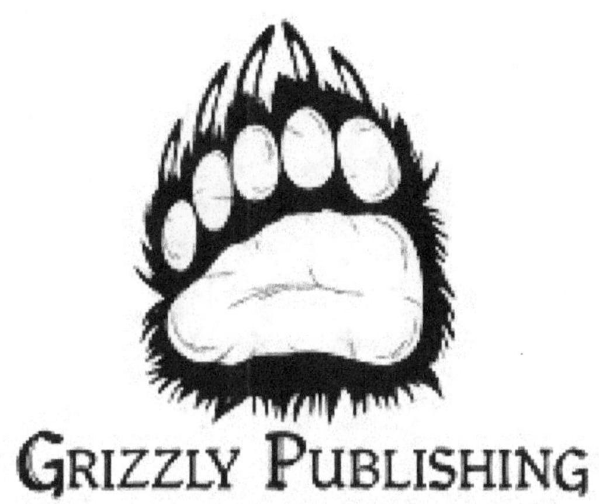

GRIZZLY PUBLISHING

www.grizzlypublishing.com

TABLE OF CONTENTS

iv

INTRODUCTION V

CHAPTER ONE: THE LAWS OF ATTRACTION 1

CHAPTER TWO: TRICKS TO BUILD LEAN MUSCLE............................6

CHAPTER THREE: EXERCISES FOR LEAN MUSCLES 11

CHAPTER FOUR: DIET TO FOLLOW 16

CHAPTER FIVE: SIMPLE RECIPES AND A MEAL PLAN 20

CHAPTER SIX: NATURAL SUPPLEMENTS TO CONSUME...................24

CHAPTER SEVEN: HEALTH BENEFITS OF WEIGHT LOSS AND MUSCLES GAIN 28

CONCLUSION 37

Introduction

I want to thank you for choosing this book, '*How to Build a Body That Attracts Beautiful Women: Forge A Masculine Physique Based on The Laws of Nature.*'

Do you wish to attract women and become the center of attention? Are you on the lookout for secrets that are sure to make any woman fall for you? Well, this book will reveal all the laws of attraction and more!

Most men do not realize that there are just a few things that they need to modify to attract women. In fact, most men already have what it takes to attract the woman of their dreams and this may only require only a little polishing.

The book details include undertaking a few exercises and making some dietary modifications that can help you develop a healthy body and mind. These are attractive qualities that appeal to most women.

Once you develop these and display confidence, women will begin to fall for you. They will be attracted to the person that you are and be drawn to your personality.

I hope you have a good time reading it and put some of the advice into practice.

Thanks again for purchasing this book. I hope you enjoy it!

Good luck!

How to Build A Body That Attracts Beautiful Women

Forge a Masculine Body that Women Can't Resist

Chapter One

The Laws of Attraction

In this first chapter of the book, we will look at some of the basics of the law of attraction. There happen to be two main theories or parameters that people consider to be laws of attraction. They are known as the halo effect and the golden ratio. These are two theories that have been tested over time and prove to be legitimate standards. So, therefore, the more a person's physical assets fit within the parameters of the golden ratio and the halo effect, the more attractive they remain.

Many psychologists have termed it as a very interesting way of looking at how science works and how evolutionary psychology plays a big role in making people think in certain ways. It is these theories that help in making up people's minds on whether someone is attractive or not.

The golden ratio is a concept that emphasizes on the perfect body shape that a man must possess to attract women. The concept is based on ideas of symmetry and how your body is structured. This does not mean that women will look at you and start calculating to check if you are attractive. But if your body fits into the parameters then you will be instantly attractive to women.

One of the parameters of the golden ratio is the waist to shoulder measurement. This ratio is used to check whether a person has the right proportions and remain attractive to women. Broad shoulders indicate strength, virility and authority and are often treated as gold standards of attraction. However, this "broad" differs from person to person and depends on the shoulder to waist ratio.

If you wish to make the most of this golden ratio, then you have to know about the Adonis index. The index is one that states your shoulders are broader than your waist. If you have such an appearance, then you will be easy to spot from anywhere and can draw in instant attraction. The perfect dimensions of this ratio are known as the golden ratio. So, say for example your waist is given the value of 1; in this case, your shoulder should be 1.618. These numbers will put you in the category of ideal Adonis axis. 1.618 is considered to be the golden number.

The right way of going about this is by measuring your waist and then developing your shoulders accordingly. It will be easier than going the other way around. So, say for example your waist measures 30 inches. Your goal will be to develop shoulders that are 48.54 inches. If you keep these parameters in mind, then you can develop the perfect body.

On the other side, if you happen to have naturally broader shoulders then you can work on reducing your waist size proportionately so that they fall within these parameters. So, if your shoulders happen to be 55 inches, then you have to develop a waist that is around 34 inches. This will be proportionate to your shoulders and make you appear attractive.

This theory proves that you do not have to be super skinny to be attractive to others. You have to bear the measurements in mind and work on your body to fall within the prescribed numbers.

Here is a simple example to help you understand how you can go about the process of fitting within the parameters.

Let's say you have a waist that is 28 inches and shoulders are 40 inches. Your current Adonis index stands at 1.43. This means that you have to put in some level of effort to change the dimensions of your body to fall within the recommended parameters.

To do this, you have to work on increasing your shoulder broadness or increase the size of your waist. You can choose either based on whatever is easier to accomplish. If you have always been skinny, then you might find it tough to modify your waist size but, through proper exercise, it might be easy to develop broad shoulder muscles.

If you consume foods that bulk your abdomen area, then you will be able to increase your waist size. Remember that you do not have to force yourself to develop perfect shoulders and waist size. It is fine if the ratio goes to 1.58 or 1.61 etc.

One of the biggest advantages associated with calculating your Adonis index and modifying your workouts is that you will know exactly what exercises to take up so that you can fall within the recommended parameters. This means that you can pick work out regimes based on how you wish to modify your body.

In fact, if you pay attention to your waist to shoulder ratio then your perfect body is extremely easy to develop and within arms reach.

Here are some pointers to get you started.

- First off, measure yourself and write it down.

- If your goal is to lose weight around the abdomen to develop the ideal waist, then pick exercises that fight fat loss. Pick exercises that will help you move your waist size to fit within the Adonis axis.

- If you wish to increase the size of your shoulders, then take up exercises that will help you in doing so.

- The basic idea is to get it to go to 1.68 times your waist measurement or a number close to it.

Once you get there, you have to put in the efforts to maintain it. You will see that it is easy to maintain your body since you will know exactly how many inches you should maintain.

Halo effect

The halo effect is another parameter that you can use to measure the attractiveness of a male. It is believed that people tend to assume that those who are attractive tend to have special, additional traits and qualities that make them attractive.

As per the halo effect, it is common for people to assume that qualities such as intelligence, productivity and success are instantly attractive to others. It is these features that people look for while looking for partners.

In fact, research studies have found that those who are attractive get more help from others compared to less attractive people and those involved in court cases receive less punishment as compared to others.

This type of phenomenon is said to happen without any conscious bearing. People do not think that they are being biased towards attractive people, it happens to be an unconscious decision. This type of attractiveness tends to cause a halo that people are blinded by and often end up making unconscious decisions.

Let us now look at what causes this attractiveness and why it is a big part of our lives.

As per psychologists, people are forced to believe that something is attractive based on what they see on television and keep in mind some parameters that they use to check whether someone is attractive or not. Say, for example, movies always portray the hero to be better looking, wealthy and always winning at the end. Most people tend to think the same way and end up like those who are attractive and good-looking.

Research studies have shown that several people who are considered attractive are also intelligent and successful. This is because intelligent and attractive people tend to find and marry their equal matches and end up having children who are intelligent and attractive. So, if you wish to attract a good-looking woman, then you must make the effort of looking good yourself.

The attractiveness of the halo effect is considered the light we tend to feel and experience in the company of others who we feel are attractive. So, if someone will make you feel great about yourself, then you have convinced yourself that they are attractive. Once you do, nothing but their good qualities will seem attractive to you.

So essentially, the more attractive you are, the higher your chances of attracting attractive women. Apart from women, you also stand the chance of attracting better jobs, higher salaries, etc. A halo is automatically created once you develop inner confidence and exude it outwards. Women will be attracted to your overall persona and take an instant liking to you.

But it is not so easy to develop a halo and takes quite a lot of effort. You should be ready to change the way you think and how you present yourself.

Chapter Two

Tricks to Build Lean Muscle

If you wish to develop a ripped body, then it is important to follow a strict diet and an exercise regime that aims to help you tone your muscles. The diet has to be such that it allows you to break your meal into 6 to 7 smaller meals so that you can digest the food easily and your body gets the right number of carbs. The exercise routine should be rigorous and make you feel the burn.

But these are well-known theories. If you wish to know about some of the secrets of building lean muscles, then read on!

Dietary cheats

You must know that a clean diet is one of the most abused diets in the world of bodybuilding. Every other builder wants to get on a clean diet to develop the body of his dreams. However, it is not important to note that you do not have to undertake a clean diet to develop a lean body. If you cheat a little, then it will prove to be advantageous for you. But this does not mean that you end up consuming processed and junk foods. It means that sometimes increasing the good fat in your diet can help you lose weight faster. The science behind this is that when you diet, the levels of leptin in your body begin to drop. Leptin keeps your hunger levels low and raises your metabolism. So, when the metabolism rises, leptin levels fall, and you burn less calories and end up eating more. When you overeat, your leptin levels get a boost, and your metabolism rises, and hunger lowers and lets you burn away more calories and consumes less food. Try to increase your daily calorie intake by 25 to 50 percent one day a week and double your carb intake on that day.

Eating before bed

When you are asleep, your body goes into a state of fasting. And ends up removing amino acids from your muscles that act as food for your brain when there is no food available. Muscle loss usually tends to negatively impact metabolism and can stand in the way of your weight loss. So, eating just before hitting the sack will meat that the amino acids are taken away from the meal and not from your muscles. But that does not mean you go only for proteins and fats. A few foods to consider include yogurt, cheese, nuts and protein powders. These happen to be slow digesting foods that can encourage your body to burn additional fat. Consuming chili and spice products that contain casein can also help you burn more of your fat. You can consume about half a cup of low-fat cottage cheese along with some chili powder or paprika. Make cutlets using them or a simple curry.

Slow carbs before workout

One mistake that most people make before going for a workout is that they tend to consume fast carbs. Although these will give you a great deal of energy, they will not help you burn away the fat as with slow digesting carbs. It is even better if they are low glycemic according to studies, those athletes who consumed a meal before working out that contains slow digesting carbs and proteins had the chance to burn away more fat when working out and during exercise in general. They were also able to keep off exhaustion for longer giving them the chance to work out more. Try to consume about 25 to 45 grams of low glycemic carbs along with about 22 grams of whey protein just before 30 minutes of working out. You can choose between oatmeal and sweet potatoes.

Fat is good

Do not make the mistake of cutting down on fat in your body. If you wish to be ripped, then it is key to incorporate some amount of fat. Some healthy fats include the likes of omega three fatty acids ad they can help you lower your body fats. Some good sources of this fat include salmon fish, olive oil, eggs and nuts. As per studies, a group of people who consumed lots of almonds was able to lose more weight and body fat as compared to those who consumed meals that contained the same number of calories and carbs but lower fats. You must try to maintain the daily calorie intake to about 20 to 30 percent per day. Consuming eggs in the morning can help you incorporate a good deal of good fat in the morning. They can help you lose a significant amount of weight as well. Consume three whole eggs followed by three egg whites.

Fruits to consume

You might not agree with me if I say that some fruits are better at helping you lose weight compared to others. This is because we tend to think of all fruits as being less calorific and having the least carbs and thus helping us lose weight faster. However, it is possible to achieve better results by consuming certain fruits as compared to others. As per study reports, people who consumed half a grapefruit and drank grapefruit juice three times a day were able to burn fat better and lost about 4 pounds of weight in 12 weeks. This can be owing to grapefruit having the ability to lower the insulin levels in the body and increase the rate of metabolism. Apples also make a great choice to lose weight as they contain antioxidants as well as boost and strengthen your body and assist with weight loss. Consume a glass of grapefruit in the mornings and have one during your evening snack and a large apple during lunch or dinner or before working out.

Calcium intake

Many people do not realize that consuming dairy is not about increasing the protein intake. It is about the calcium intake that can greatly help with weight loss. Calcium is known to help with weight loss, especially from the ab area. It is believed that a hormone known as calcitriol helps in gaining fat and slows down the burning of fat. When calcium is consumed, this hormone is suppressed to a great extent thereby allowing you to lose more weight. Calcium can also reduce the level of dietary fat that is consumed and absorbed by your intestines and might also lower your appetite. Go for dairy products that are low in fat such as Greek yogurt and skimmed milk. Consume them at least twice a day, as they will also enhance the level of proteins in your body.

Go for organics

It is important to consume organically grown produce even if it means shelling out a little extra. If you care about your health, then it is important to consume all-natural food products that are good for your body. As per a study, those who consumed organic milk ended up consuming 70 percent more omega three fats compared to those who consumed regular milk. Those who consumed organic meats had more omega three fatty acids that help in burning away fats and building lean muscles. So, try to go for organic milk, cottage cheese and eggs as much as possible.

Consume cold water

It is understood that drinking water can help you in greatly reducing your body fat. But one neat trick is to consume cold water, which can greatly help you in losing weight and developing lean muscles. As per studies, those who consumed 2 cups of cold water had the chance to enhance metabolic activity by 30%. It is known that this is due to an increase in the norepinephrine levels that is brought on by the consumption of water. According to another study, those who drank 2 cups of water in between meals consumed less food and lost more weight compared to those who did not drink any water in between meals. So, you must drink about 2 cups of water during your meals so that you can digest the food better.

Many people are used to consuming sodas and artificially sweetened drinks that end up adding unnecessary calories. Research shows that they also tend to increase your appetite and might cause you to consume more food than your body needs. It is best to avoid drinking these and depend on water to lose weight faster.

Consume soy

Most men trying to lose weight and develop muscles do not think of soya as something they should add to their diet. However, it is important to consume soya if you wish to develop lean muscles. Soya is a natural fat burner that burns away fat at a rapid pace. Research has found that those who consume 20 grams of soya per day can lose quite a lot of weight, especially in the abdominal area as compared to consuming foods containing casein. Soya helps in building lean muscles and increase the level of growth hormones in the body. Try to consume at least 10 grams of soy protein per day.

Chapter Three

Exercises for Lean Muscles

If you wish to develop a healthy and lean body, then you have to take up an exercise routine that is designed to help you lose weight and maintain lean muscles.

There is a misconception that it is not possible to pick exercises that can help you develop muscles as well as slim you down. However, if you choose the right blend of exercises, then you can see faster results and get more from your workouts.

If you wish to lose weight faster then you can take up the lean mass 15 routine that happens to be a month-long fitness plan. It is used to develop lean muscles and increase cardio while burning away the fat. It is a high-intensity routine that can help you build muscles faster.

Since it is high intensity, it is not an exercise plan that can be followed for more than four weeks. You can take this up for a month and then go back to your routine to lose weight. You might also have to take a small break to help your body recuperate. If you go about continuously exercising, then it will end up stressing you out.

Once you decide to take up this routine, you have to prepare yourself to take up more physical activities and rest little. Your rest periods will also include some form of activities so that your body is in constant motion. So, you will be giving your body a complete and thorough work out that can help you reduce the fat content in your body at a rapid pace.

This exercise program is pretty easy to follow and can be modified to suit your body type. You can pack in maximum activity in minimum time. It is effective in reducing fat and increasing lean muscles.

When you wish to develop stronger muscles, you have to be able to do an exercise repeatedly for long periods of times or a larger number of repetitions. Then, and only then, will you be able to achieve the desired results. For example, a person who does a higher number of squats during a work out regime has the chance to burn away more fat and develop stronger muscles as compared to someone who does less squats. So, the key is to train your muscles to become stronger and not burn away easily. However, stronger muscles do not mean they are leaner, and so, you have to ensure that the exercises you take up target the right muscles.

Here are some exercises that target the waist.

Side Planks

- Lie down on the floor balancing your body on the left side. Place a rolled-up towel between your thighs.

- Your forearm has to be perpendicular to your torso.

- Your foot should be on the floor in front of your left foot to support your base.

- Lift up your hips such that your body remains in a straight line from your head to your toe and squeeze the towel tightly between your thighs. Hold it there and count until 60.

- Repeat this ten times and do three sets of it.

Fly ups

- Sit down on a mat on the floor and lean backward to place your elbow and legs together over a wall such that your knees bend at 90 degrees.

- Raise your legs upwards and lean them against the wall and then press your lower back on to the floor and squeeze your abs as you raise arms to reach your feet. Keep your elbows soft.

- Press your feet into the wall.

- Curl up about 1 inch and do 20 pulses. Come down about an inch.

- Do three sets of this and keep trying to touch your knees to your chest.

Twisted curl

- Sit on the floor and bend your knees and lay down your feet flat on the ground.

- Rest your elbows on the floor.

- Press your lower back on the floor and squeeze your abs together and curl up your torso towards the left side. Lift your arms such that your hands hold the left thigh.

- Holding the curl position, you have to gently free your hands such that they move to the outside of your thigh and do 20 push-ups.

- Curl up your torso to the left by an inch and then lower it by an inch. Place your hands on your thighs for pulse rate.

- Raise your arms up and keep switching the sides. Do three sets of this exercise.

Shoulder widening exercises

Side lateral raise

- Pick out dumbbells that you would like to use and stand with your torso straight and the dumbbells on your side at arm's length and the palms facing you as the starting position.

- Hold your torso still and lift up the dumbbells towards your sides with a slight bend on the elbow and your hands slightly tilted to look like you are pouring water. Keep going up until your arms are parallel to the floor.

- Exhale your breath and stop for a second once your arms reach the top.

- Bring down the dumbbells to a certain position as you take a breath.

- Do this for the remaining reps.

Angled dumbbell side raise

- Choose dumbbells that you will be using for this exercise. Stand up straight and hold the dumbbells to your side at arm's length with your palms facing you. This should be the starting position.

- Stay stationary in your starting position and lift the dumbbells to your side by bending your elbow a little and keeping your hands forward.

- Hold the pose once you reach the top.

- Bring the dumbbell down and inhale.

- Repeat for the remaining reps.

Standing straight sidebar raise

- Pick dumbbells that you will use for this exercise. Your non-lifting hand should be used to hold on to something that is steady to help you gain support.

- Now lean towards your lifting arm and keep it away from the hand that is gripping the bench as it can help you balance your body.

- Hold on to the bench tightly and raise your dumbbell to the side. Keep lifting it until it is parallel to the floor.

- Breathe in when lowering and breathe out while lifting the dumb bell.

- Repeat for the recommended reps.

Apart from these, there are many other exercises that you can take up. Some yoga poses can be performed after your cardio and strengths training. You can pick poses that help with toning down the abs and strengthening the shoulders.

Chapter Four

Diet to Follow

Building a healthy body requires you to take on the right form of exercises as well as maintain a nutritious and healthy diet. We already looked at some dietary tricks to adopt and, in this chapter, we will look at some of the best foods to consume when trying to lose weight and develop lean muscles.

Beef

Beef is one of the most important lean muscles to add to your diet owing to the protein content, the cholesterol, zinc and iron that is present in it. These are required to develop a lean body and stronger muscles. Try to go for organic beef meat or grass-fed beef. They will have higher levels of conjugated linoleic acid or CLA compared to commercially grown cattle. This type of fat helps you shed fat and muscles easily.

Beetroots

Beetroots are a rich source of a chemical known as Betaine or trimethylglycine that is used to enhance liver health as well as joint health. Beetroots also help in increasing muscle power and help you carry out exercises better. Consuming beetroots after your workout can help you recover faster.

Brown rice

Brown rice is a whole grain that is slowly digested by the body. It helps in providing energy for a longer period that can last you all throughout your exercise routine. Replace your regular rice with brown rice to fight away the fight much easier.

Orange

A good fruit to consider adding to your daily intake is orange. Oranges are full of antioxidants and can enhance your strength and endurance. You can consume one orange before your workouts.

Cantaloupes

Cantaloupes are a great choice to consume when trying to lose weight, as they are low in fructose content. It is preferred to melons and can be consumed in the mornings during breakfast. You can also have it before hitting the gym.

Cottage cheese

Cottage cheese is a great addition to your diet. It is a rich source of protein and can be consumed before going to bed. You can make your cottage cheese at home if you think the ones in the market are not organic. By consuming it at night, the catabolism during sleep can be prevented.

Eggs

Eggs are a great source of protein and can help you feel fuller for longer periods of time. Eat them in the morning and for lunch. They will give you a boost of proteins and keep you energetic throughout the day or work out regime.

Milk

You must consume organic milk that contains whey protein and casein. It is rich in amino acids such as glutamine. It contains a lot more omega three fatty acids and can help you increase your overall health.

Quinoa

Quinoa is full of proteins and is a slow digesting carb. Quinoa helps in increasing the insulin levels in your body. It is best to consume when you wish to develop leaner muscles and gain overall strength.

Spinach

Spinach contains glutamine, which is an amino acid that is required to grow lean muscles and has lots of antioxidants. These antioxidants will reduce cell damage and assist in improving your overall health.

Apples

Apples are a rich source of polyphenols that can increase muscle endurance and help you last longer in the gym. You can take up exercises for a longer period. You can have an apple in the morning and one before your workout.

Greek yogurt

There is nothing better than Greek yogurt to meet a large portion of your daily protein and calcium intake. It has a lot more protein compared to regular yogurt. It also has lesser carbs and happens to be a good source of casein proteins. Have at least 2 cups per day and avoid flavored ones.

Whole wheat bread

Consume bread that is made using organic whole wheat. It contains grains that are rich in proteins and contain amino acids. It can help with lean muscle growth. Replace your regular white flour bread with whole wheat bread.

Wheat germ

Wheat germ is rich in nutrients such as selenium, zinc, and iron as well as potassium and B vitamins. It also contains amino acids and glutamine that is good for the body. The high levels of fiber content in wheat germ make it ideal for everyday consumption. Wheat germ is a slow digestive carbohydrate and can be consumed before going to bed and before workouts.

Chapter Five

Simple Recipes and a Meal Plan

Here are some simple diet recipes to prepare.

Diet Chicken Curry

Ingredients:

- 2 Onions, chopped

- 2 Garlic cloves, chopped

- 2 chilies, chopped

- 1-inch ginger, grated

- 500 grams no fat, skinned chicken breasts

- five tablespoons fat-free Greek yogurt

- 1 teaspoon cumin seeds

- 1 teaspoon coriander seeds powder

- 1 teaspoon turmeric powder

- Salt to taste

- 1 teaspoon Indian curry powder

- 2 cans tomatoes, chopped

- 1 teaspoon vegetable oil or coconut oil

Recipe:

1. Chop the onion, garlic, and ginger finely and slit the chilies.

2. Add them to a blender and whizz until smooth.

3. Add it to a bowl along with the yogurt and mix until well combined.

4. Add the chicken and mix well.

5. Allow it to marinate for an hour or two.

6. Add oil to a saucepan and heat it.

7. Add the chicken pieces and fry it on both sides.

8. Add the chopped tomatoes in along with salt, Indian curry powder, cumin seeds, turmeric and coriander powder and mix until well combined.

9. Add little water and cover to cook for 10 minutes.

10. Serve warm.

Cottage Cheese Salad

Ingredients:

- 1 cup low fat cottage cheese

- 1 large tomato, chopped

- 1/2 cup cucumber, chopped

- 1/3 cup green pepper, chopped

- 2 tablespoons mayonnaise, low fat

- 1 tablespoon sour cream, low fat

- 1 tablespoon low-fat salsa

- Cilantro leaves to sprinkle

Recipe:

1. Crumble the cottage cheese into a bowl.

2. Add the chopped tomatoes and cucumber along with the bell peppers and toss.

3. Add the mayonnaise and sour cream and salsa and toss.

4. Serve with a sprinkling of cilantro leaves on top.

Meal plan

Here is a simple meal plan that you can follow for a month or two to see a difference in your physique.

Breakfast 1

Start your day with a scoop of whey protein added to a glass of skimmed or low-fat milk and consume half a muskmelon.

Breakfast 2

After about 30 minutes to an hour of consuming breakfast 1, you must consume breakfast 2. Consume 3 large eggs in the form of omelet or scramble along with 2 slices of low-fat ham and ¼ cup of cheddar cheese. You can also consume a cup of cooked oatmeal.

Morning snack

Consume 4 ounces of Greek yogurt that has reduced fat. Follow up with half a cup of blueberries.

Lunch

4 ounces lean ground beef, 1 whole-wheat burger bun, 2 cups of mixed green beans and 1-tablespoon olive oil and balsamic vinegar.

Mid-day snack

3 ounces of low-fat chicken used to make curry (recipe provided) or salad, 1 tablespoon lightly beaten mayonnaise, 5 whole-wheat crackers.

Dinner

6 ounces turkey breasts cooked and added to salads or curries. 1-cup broccoli steamed, 2 cups mixed greens such as spinach and kale and green beans tossed with a tomato salad and dressed with a tablespoon of olive oil.

Night Snack

¾ cup cottage cheese curry or salad along with 2 tablespoons tomato salsa as dressing. (Recipe provided)

Chapter Six

Natural Supplements to Consume

If you wish to develop a healthy body then here are some natural supplements to consider. These natural supplements can increase the rate at which you burn fat and develop the body of your dreams.

Chitosan

Chitosan is sugar that is found in the outer layers of seafood such as shrimps and crabs. According to scientists, this sugar can block fats and cholesterol from being absorbed into your skin and make its way to your body. Although there has not been enough research on this topic, it is believed that Chitosan helps in cutting down on body fats to some extent and helps with digestion. Chitosan does not have any known side effects. You can get this chemical into your systems by consuming seafood such as lobsters and crabs.

Chromium picolinate

Chromium happens to be a mineral that helps in enhancing insulin function in the body. It is a hormone that is essential to turn food into energy. Our bodies require chromium to convert and store the carbs, fats, and proteins. As per studies, chromium can be consumed to reduce the appetite, burn away calories and cut down on body fats. It also helps in increasing the muscle mass.

But make sure you consume within the recommended limits as otherwise, it can lead to insomnia, headaches, etc.

Ashwagandha

Ashwagandha has been used in traditional Indian medicine for thousands of years. It is known to cut down on the fat content in the body and promotes weight loss. It is a natural adaptogen and has been proven to fight away stress. Consuming just a little amount can help you maintain a calm mind and develop a strong body. Ashwagandha capsules and tablets are quite popular around the world and used for stress relief and weight loss.

Ginseng

Ginseng is a Chinese herb that is used to fight away excess fat and develop a slim body. It can boost your energy levels and keep you going throughout the day. It helps with regulating blood sugar levels thereby ensuring that your diabetes is under control. Ginseng root and root powder are available online and can be consumed. But make sure it is genuine and buy only from trusted dealers.

Ginkgo Biloba

Ginkgo Biloba is an herb that is consumed to increase blood flow to cells. It has been used in Chinese medicine for hundreds of years. It is still extremely popular and used in the weight loss industry. It is also consumed for its high antioxidant content. Ginkgo also helps to increase the level of testosterone in the body. It can be consumed in powdered and tablet form.

CLA

CLA is known as conjugated linoleic acid. It is a popular supplement that is present in fatty acids called linoleic acid. It helps to control body fat and helps you remain full. As per research, CLA helps in losing weight and enhancing muscle gain. Just by consuming 2 grams of CLA you can effectively control weight loss and increase muscle mass. However, you have to consult your physician first as some of its side effects include insulin resistance and nausea.

Green tea extract

Green tea is a popular supplement that has been consumed since time immemorial. It helps in curbing the appetite and enhancing metabolism. Green tea is full of antioxidants that are required to keep you healthy and helps in fighting away oxidative damage. Apart from drinking green tea regularly, it is also important for you to consume green tea supplements. However, do not drink tea too close to bedtime as it can lead to insomnia.

Green coffee

According to research, it is possible to lose weight by consuming green coffee extracts. Green coffee extract can help in cutting down on the fat content in your body and accelerate metabolism. Green coffee extract can be consumed in the form of powder or capsule.

Guar gum

Guar gum is a fiber-rich supplement that can be consumed to enhance digestive capacity. It is helpful in dissolving fats in the body. Guar gum helps you feel full and cut down on your appetite to a large extent. Guar gum can be consumed in powder form on a daily basis.

Hoodia

Hoodia is a plant that grows in the desserts of Africa. It has been used by tribal folk since time immemorial to cut down on their hunger during long trips. Hoodia is now consumed as an appetite suppressant to control hunger. It contains a chemical known as P57 that helps in controlling hunger. It can be consumed in powder or tablet form.

Keto DHEA

Keto DHEA is a chemical that is naturally present in your body. It can help you lose weight and boost your metabolic activity. With the help of the chemical, you can enhance calorie burn. According to studies, people who consumed the supplement and undertook moderate exercises were able to lose a significant amount of weight. But research is still on to understand how it works and how it can help in building a fit body. But it is important to consume in the recommended dose to ensure that your body gets the right amount and does not lead to side effects.

Remember that you have to consult your physician before choosing any of these to ensure that they are safe to be consumed. If you suffer from an illness, then make sure you tell your doctor about the same and also tell him about any medicines that you currently consume.

Chapter Seven

Health Benefits of Weight Loss and Muscles Gain

When it comes to weight loss, there are many different benefits that your body will receive. In this chapter, we will look at them in detail and also look at how you can increase the level of testosterone in your body.

Testosterone

Testosterone is a male hormone that is responsible for the development of male sexual characteristics. Testosterone helps a man develop confidence and become a leader. It is important for the male body to have enough testosterone at all times. But lifestyle choices and stress often end up depleting the level of testosterone in the body. Here are some things that can promote testosterone production in your body.

Weight loss

If you happen to be obese or overweight then losing the excess pounds can help you increase the level of testosterone in your body. Men who are overweight tend to have lower levels of testosterone in their bodies. So, it becomes important to lose weight to maintain the ideal levels of testosterone.

If you are keen on losing weight to develop a healthy body and naturally increase the level of testosterone, then it is essential to cut out as much sugar from your meals as possible. Not many men realize that sugar can be in the form of fructose and refined sugars found in processed and junk foods. So, it is essential to cut out junk and processed foods from the diet so that it is easier to lose weight. It is best to say no to sweeteners as well as they too might not be fully free from calories.

Try to consume less than 25 grams of fructose per day. If you happen to be insulin resistant, then reduce this even further.

Apart from eliminating fructose from your diet, you must also get rid of gluten-rich foods such as grains and lactose-rich foods such as raw milk. Lactose has been known to increase insulin and in turn body weight.

Try to cut out all refined carbs from your diets such as cereals; waffles, biscuits, cakes and other such foods that can contain refined white flour. They can instantly spike up your insulin levels and lead to health issues. It can also lead to weight gain and digestive issues.

You have to increase intake of healthy fats such as vegetable-based fats and grains. You can consume natural saturated fats as well. Your body should get carbs in the form of vegetables that are rich in micronutrients instead of grains as it slows down the conversion to simple sugars such as glucose and brings down the level of insulin in your body. Once you cut out the grains, you have to increase the intake of vegetables to balance it out. Go for the ones that are rich in proteins and healthy fats such as yam, artichokes, kale, spinach, beetroots, carrots, etc.

Once you switch up your diet and start losing excess pounds, your testosterone levels will automatically rise and make you a confident person.

High-intensity exercises

High-intensity exercises can help in increasing the testosterone levels in your body. Along with intermittent fasting, it can greatly help in boosting testosterone levels and help you live a healthy life.

Short and intense exercises have been proven to have a positive effect on your testosterone levels and can prevent it from going down. This is unlike other forms of exercises such as aerobics and moderate level exercises that can lead to a fall in the level of testosterone in your body.

Intermittent fasting is all about boosting the testosterone level by increasing the satiety of leptin and a group of hormones including glucagon-like peptide and melanocortins that help in the generation of healthy levels of testosterone in the body and increase the level of libido. It also helps in preventing age-related decline in the testosterone levels.

Consuming whey proteins after your workouts can help in increasing the level of testosterone in your body.

Here is a look at high-intensity exercise routine.

- Warm up for 5 minutes by stretching your body and doing a few jumping jacks.

- Indulge in intensive body exercises for the next 30 seconds and take a small break for 10 seconds before exercising again.

- Take a break after a minute and a half.

- Do this for 7 to 8 times more.

This means that you work out for only around 15 to 20 minutes per day and that will be enough to help with the increase of testosterone levels in your body.

You can do these exercises without the need for any equipment. If you want, you can be on the treadmill for 30 minutes or swim for 30 minutes to add to your exercise regime. But make sure you do not strain your body after the high-intensity exercises.

There are many types of intermittent fasts to choose from, and you can choose whatever suits you best. The 24 hours fast requires that you not consume a meal for 24 hours. The 16 hours fast requires you to not eat for 16 hours etc.

Try to consume at least eight glasses of water per day and drink fruit infused water if you are bored of regular water.

Zinc

Zinc happens to be an important nutrient to consume when you wish to lose weight as well as increase the level of testosterone in your body. Zinc helps in supplementing your diet and has been known to help in increasing testosterone content within 4 to 6 weeks. Research has shown that diets that restrict the intake of zinc can cause a drop in the level of testosterone in the body. It is therefore recommended to consume zinc tablets in case your diet does not incorporate enough zinc in it.

If you are a youngster aged 25 to 35, then it is a must that you consume foods that are rich in zinc. Your diet should also contain protein-rich foods such as meats and fish and vegetables and fruits, some natural sources of zinc include raw milk, cheese, beans, and yogurt. Meat eaters will find it easier to meet their daily zinc requirements as compared to vegetarians. So, it is important to consume larger quantities of vegetables that contain meat.

It is best to go for organic foods that have been grown naturally. Inorganically grown vegetables and fruits can have lots of chemicals that will reduce the level of zinc and prevent it from reaching your body.

You have to be careful with the way you cook your food and ensure that the nutrients remain intact. Make use of a slow cooker that cooks food at a lower temperature for longer periods of time.

If you plan on consuming zinc supplements, then it has to be less than 40 grams per day. If you take too much, then you might suffer from nausea.

Strength training

Apart from high-intensity training, it is also important for you to undertake strength training. It helps in boosting the level of testosterone in your body give you practice training consistently. When you take up strength training to boost your levels of testosterone, you have to increase the weight and reduce the reps and focus on exercises that work on muscles such as squats.

When you lower the pace and movement, you end up converting it into high-intensity exercises. Slow movement helps your muscles and can help you grow leaner muscles that are tougher to lose.

Vary the weights that you use to train and ensure that you make it progressively heavier.

Vitamin D

It is important to increase the vitamin D intake to develop healthy nucleus in sperm cells. Vitamin D also helps in boosting sperm count in your body. Vitamin D enhances testosterone levels and boosts libido. As per one study, those who were overweight were given vitamin D supplements saw a spike in their levels of testosterone within a single year.

Vitamin D deficiency is now quite common, as people do not spend enough time in the sun. So, chances are, you are by default having a vitamin D deficiency, and so, you have to consume a supplement that can replenish the nutrient in your body.

You can visit your doctor to get a test done to determine how much vitamin D you have and what supplement can be consumed to fix it. You must have between 50 to 70 ng/ml.

A good way to naturally increase the levels is by spending as much time in the sun as possible. Try to be out in the sun for at least 30 minutes and catch the morning sun. Your skin should turn light pink. Take up a sport so that you can be out in the sun as well as get some exercise.

Cut down on stress

Stressing out too much can negatively impact your body's testosterone levels. When you undertake stress, your body ends up releasing a hormone known as cortisol. Cortisol can end up blocking the level of testosterone that is produced and released into your body. This is because cortisol is a chemical that is released to combat a stressful situation or an emergency and testosterone are used for sexual activity, confidence, etc. and not considered to be an emergency hormone.

Modern day lifestyles have known to cause a rapid depletion in the level of testosterone in the body. This is because of the presence of immense cortisol that is brought on by daily stress. So, the most important thing to do is to cut down on day-to-day stress so that it is easier for your body to produce the right amounts of testosterone.

There are many natural techniques that you can use to reduce stress. Some of them include taking up meditation, yoga, indulging in a hobby, etc. if these are not working and you seem to have immense stress, you can take up acupressure or stress-reducing massages to help you out.

There are many types of meditational practices to pick from and here are some of them.

- Breathing meditation is one of the most practiced forms of meditation. Close your eyes and sit in a quiet place. Focus on your breath and visualize it going into your lungs and exiting. This will help you calm down.

- Chanting meditation is one where you sit down in a comfortable position and chant a calming word. The word should resonate with your body and vibrate as you chant.

- Visualization is a technique that is used to help people get over a stressful situation. All you have to do is think of a future situation where you visualize yourself as having conquered all your issues and leading a great life. You can also visualize yourself surrounded by attractive and successful women who are attracted to you.

Certain habits such as smoking and doing drugs can increase stress levels. You have to stay away from these habits if you wish to increase the testosterone level in your body.

No sugar!

As a rule, you have to cut out all possible sources of sugar from your diet if you wish to develop a healthy body. As per research studies, testosterone levels tend to go down drastically after consuming sugar. Sugar can cause a drop in insulin levels, therefore, leading to lower levels of testosterone in the body.

According to estimates, an average American consumes 12 teaspoons of sugar every day, which is about two whole tons for a lifetime.

Sugar happens to be like a drug that tends to make you happy by increasing the dopamine levels in your brain. You are drawn to consuming more sugar just to feel good. So, it becomes important to resist its consumption and cut down on sugar in your diet.

Once you get into the habit of consuming foods containing sugar on a regular basis, you will find it quite difficult to get off the habit. It is therefore important to avoid consuming sugar-based foods. Fructose is another plant-based sugar that can negatively impact your health. Cut out fructose from your diet as well so that you can make the most of your diet.

Healthy Fats

Healthy fats are great for your body and can help you maintain and increase testosterone levels. Healthy fats such as polyunsaturated and monounsaturated fats are found in avocados and nuts and are extremely important when you wish to increase the level of testosterone levels in your body.

According to experts, it is best to consume about 70 percent fat per meal. It is essential to know that your body needs saturated fats that can be availed through animal and vegetables such as oils, coconut and meats. Try to avoid consuming vegetables that are rich in carbs and go for the ones that contain natural and healthy oils.

BCAA

Research has shown that BCAA can result in the production of higher testosterone in the body when consumed and coupled with resistance training. BCAAs are available in the form of supplements and can be found in higher concentrations in dairy products. They are highest in whey proteins and cheeses.

Leucine that is found in natural foods is often wasted as a base instead of an anabolic agent. So, to have the right anabolic environment, one has to increase leucine content in the body and maintain higher levels.

Bear in mind that leucine consumed as a free forming amino acid can work against your cause when free form amino acid is consumed as they can disrupt insulin activity in the bloodstream. It can impair the glycemic control in your body. It is best to consume this chemical in the form of food-based leucine as it can help you develop leaner, stronger muscles and avoid the side effects.

Conclusion

I thank you again for choosing this book and hope you had a good time reading it.

The main aim of this book was to educate you on the basics of using the golden ratio and the halo effect to attract women.

If you put the advice in this book to practice, then you can develop a healthy mind and body. It is important to build a lean body to maintain good health and increase productivity. Use the diet tips to consume healthier meals and give yourself the advantage of leading a longer and healthier life.

I wish you luck and hope you develop the body of your dreams.

Finally, if you enjoyed this book then I'd like to ask you for a favor. Will you be kind enough to leave a review for this book on Amazon? It would be greatly appreciated!

Thank you and good luck!

Other Books by Grizzly Publishing

3 Book Australian Travel Bundle: How To Pack Your Bag When Traveling to Australia, Hostels Shopping: Checklist On Traveling Australia In Hostels & Flight Hacking: Learn The Secrets To Flying For Free

https://www.amazon.com/dp/B07C8FH4X9

How to Pack Your Bag When Traveling to Australia: Backpackers Essential Item List

https://www.amazon.com/dp/B077NY71TM

How To Teach English Overseas: Use Your Native Language To Fund Your Travels All Over The World

https://www.amazon.com/dp/B078K9FNGY

Ketogenic Diet for Beginners: Step by Step Instructions to Embracing the Keto Lifestyle

https://www.amazon.com/dp/B077GS49J3

Beijing In 72 Hours: Maximize Your Layover With Our 3 Day Plan

https://www.amazon.com/dp/B078XDBSRC